# Why America Is Fat,

## The Truth Is Finally Revealed!

## Rino Soriano

### Disclaimer

This book is designed to provide information on holistic health living. It is distributed with the understanding that the author and publisher are not engaged in rendering medical advice or medical claims about your health and well-being. Rino is not a licensed health practitioner or doctor. He is an educator in holistic health and has experience in holistic nutrition, fitness, and supplemental health programs.

Every effort has been made to make this manual complete and as accurate as possible. However, there may be errors in both typographical and content. Therefore, this text should be used as a general guide and not the ultimate source for improving your health. Furthermore, this manual contains holistic health information that is current only up to the printing date.

The main intent of this manual is to educate and entertain. BodyBuilding Brilliance and the author and publisher Flying Hawk Productions, LLC shall have neither liability nor responsibility to any person or entity with respect to any loss or damage caused by or allegedly to have been caused, directly or indirectly, by the information in this book.

# Table of Contents

# Chapter 1

## Are You Ready To Get Off The Hamster Wheel???

Hi there my friend, are you ready to learn the holistic pathway for being healthy and slim? I am sure you are, as the many so called weight reduction solutions and health paradigms out there simply have not and do not validate themselves with results that last.

It is quite obvious that these so called solutions are not effective for most people for reducing their weight and keeping it off. There are valid reasons why and if you allow me to introduce some holistic principles for health and for being slim then I think you will fare much better than you have with all of the diets and erroneous health information out there.

Are you ready to get your world rocked? All I ask is that you leave an open mind and use your heart to see if what I teach resonates with you and if you feel it is true. I teach holistic principles that validate themselves as they honor nature and the unique multi-dimensional constitution of a human being.

Most health paradigms are attempting to teach you a one size fits all. As has been proven by millions of people worldwide...**you cannot standardize health and put it into a box and then serve all people with this one paradigm.** That is erroneous once you truly comprehend the holistic science of a human body and the True makeup of each person.

I think you get my main point here. If all of the current health paradigms out there are valid then you would have millions of people by now that would be slim and healthy. However, we now have more overweight and unhealthy people than ever before. Yet, there is more health information out there than ever before. So, what gives? Why do most health paradigms do not help people to be healthy and slim and radiant? I will get into that as you go through this ebook on Holistic Slimming as I teach.

First, is that you must learn the True Holistic Science of your body and what it Truly requires for optimum health. It is your responsibility to learn how to care for your health and well-being. Do you really think that someone else can tell you how to be healthy and slim??? My friend, millions of people have gone to that approach and the results speak for themselves. You are the only one that knows what is best for your health and well-being with some guidance from your intuition and your body wisdom. These are your best reflectors of how to care for your health.

It is time for you to wake up and take your power and learn the holistic pathway to being slim and healthy. Conventional health paradigms have had more than enough time to validate themselves and again the results speak for themselves.

So, let me begin to lay a holistic foundation for you so that you may elevate your consciousness as to see the Truth of why so many people are overweight and unhealthy these days. I call it holistic science as it honors nature and Universal Life Principles that you can observe and apply in your life and the results speak for themselves.

## Chapter 2

### Eating Fat Does Not Make You Make Fat

Ok, please listen up. The common health paradigms that say eating fat makes you fat is so erroneous. Where this came from I have no idea, however, it is not based on holistic science. Let me clarify for you why this erroneous philosophy is not true. First of all, is that everything you ingest gets broken down by the body into smaller components at a molecular level. For instance, if you ingest protein, the body breaks it down into smaller components called amino acids. This is the only way your body can make use of the protein you ingested.

So, in the instance of fat, your body also breaks this down into smaller components called lipids. Actually, when you ingest fat the body breaks it down into 2 components. The one is water and the other is lipid molecules. Again, your body has to transform fat into these base elements in order for them to be absorbed by your system. Once this happens the fat you ingested is no longer fat as you know of it. It is a new structure of nutrient that your body takes in as hydration and energy. **Eating any fat is not going to translate into that fat being stored anywhere on your body as many people have been led to believe.** This is a myth my friend!

So, as you can see now the common health paradigms that say eating fat makes you fat is super erroneous. **Ingesting fat does not make you fat, never has, never will.** What will make you gain weight is by ingesting the wrong ratios of foods, sugar foods, processed foods and any foods that are not meant to go in the human body.

**Healthy fats are the most essential nutrients your body requires to be healthy. Healthy fats are also the greatest source of energy for your body.**

There are certain types of foods that will alter your metabolism and cause you weight gain. There are many that will do this and most people are ingesting these foods that are not meant to go in the human body. As such, you can see in society what ingesting the wrong kinds of nutrition has done to a majority of the population. The proof is in the pudding my friend. I am simply speaking holistic science here. What I teach is foundational holistic body science and yet most people have no clue of what these principles are for being slim and healthy.

As you go through this book I will teach you the foundational holistic science that you require to embody if you truly desire to be healthy and slim and radiant.

So, weight gain has very little to do with calories and fat grams. **If your body is functioning at optimal levels then weight gain will not be an issue.** However, due to the misinformation out there, most people have no clue as to how to even begin to structure their nutrition to help their body be at optimum functioning. As such, you have a weight gain issue in life.

A majority of society is programmed with erroneous information about health and wellness. Again, one look at society and there is the proof. Go to any public shopping center and simply observe and there you will see just how many people are overweight and out of shape. It really should not be this way.

However, the current health paradigms are part of the issue. Many of these health paradigms are teaching philosophies and practices that actually are counter health and can actually make people gain weight. Again, you must come to comprehend the holistic science of your body. Once you do then this is when you can begin to embody the holistic lifestyle that will get you results that last.

There is no need to count calories and reduce your fat intake as many health paradigms teach. In fact, this is very unhealthy if you learn what your body truly requires for optimum health. This practice will put your body in survival mode since it takes a number of calories and fat to sustain your health. This approach to weight reduction is counter health for most people as it will eventually cause your body to alter the metabolism to burn calories slower.

So, some people who have done this approach may have lost a few pounds at first, however, what they lost was actually water and then if anything else they lost muscle which is the last thing you want to do for health. This is what all of the weight reduction paradigms out there are teaching and again look at what that has gotten people. You will not lose much fat, if at all, by following the limit your fat and calories approach. It is not wise or healthy nor is it required.

Limiting fat and calories from your diet will cause your body to go into survival mode because it will think you are not able to ingest the proper amounts of nutrition each day. Thus, it alters your basal metabolic rate to burn calories slower as to help keep you alive and functioning. This is a Divine protection mechanism as to help you live in case you do not have access to food for a while.

It is a holistic fact that ingesting the right kinds of healthy fats in balance can actually help you to stay slim and healthy. Healthy fats will help your metabolism to function properly and stay in balance. There are 2 main types of fat that your body requires for optimum health. One type of fat is **simple unsaturated fats** that come from primarily plants and seeds. The other type of essential fat your body requires for optimum health is **saturated**

**fat** and is actually the most important for your health.

**What most people are unaware of is that healthy saturated fats are a precursor to hormone production for your body.** These saturated fats come primarily from animal fats and are considered the KING of fats since they are so essential for human health. This means that your body requires these building compounds as to be able to produce the various number of hormones to be in homeostasis and in healthy levels.

Scientifically speaking we humans are considered animals and therefore our bodies are designed to be nourished via animal fats and protein. In case you do not know, is that there is a food chain on this planet and you require honoring nature and the Universal laws set on this domain. Many people are unaware that a human body is designed to be nourished mainly via healthy and balanced animal proteins and saturated fats. The healthiest cultures to ever walk the planet ingested high amounts of healthy saturated fats and healthy proteins.

The Eskimos were and are the healthiest group of people to ever walk the planet. Do you want to know what they ingest? They do super high quantities of raw animal milk, pure raw whale blubber, and naturally raw and fermented meats. They do virtually little starch foods as their environment does have those groups of foods available and they never consume any form of processed sugar or fruit.

Just so you know is that it is the sugary and starchy foods are lowering people's health and well-being the most of any food items. This has been proven for many decades. In fact, if you want more conclusive evidence of the ideal nutrition intake for humans then simply research Weston A Price and his discoveries. Simply looking at the photos he took of various people around the planet and what they ingested will give you a new perspective on holistic nutrition. His discoveries beyond validate that the cultures doing mainly pure wholesome foods from Mother Earth in their natural forms and super high fat and high quality animal proteins create super radiant health. Also, he discovered that the cultures that ingest any form of processed sugars or high starch foods always had health conditions and lowered health levels.

**My message to you is that if you simply observe nature and life, then you will always be shown the Truth.** Life is your greatest teacher and your greatest validator. If you want to know if something is True, then simply observe and let life show you. If you simply take a look at the common health paradigms out there, they have beyond proven that they DO NOT work well for helping humanity to be healthy, slim and radiant, not even close my friend. Begin to use a Higher Consciousness and let life show you the path to Truth.

The common health paradigms have been teaching you to reduce or remove saturated fats from your diet. You have been conditioned to think that saturated fats cause low level health. **Well, the holistic science fact is that saturated fats are KING as far as nutrients go.** They are the powerhouse of building compounds for your body and for your health to thrive. This can be validated by ingesting a balance of saturated fats for a few days and then letting your body tell you the Truth.

By reducing saturated fats from your diet, you set yourself up for low level health and improper functioning of your metabolism since your metabolism is governed by hormones. Do you see the connection? Be aware that every single biological process is governed by hormones.

So, it is counter-productive to follow the common health paradigms that say to limit your fat intake to reduce your weight. You can actually reduce your weight much easier by ingesting healthy fats (both unsaturated and saturated) on a daily basis according to your unique body constitution. This is something you must learn by beginning to incorporate holistic nutrition as I teach. When you do follow this holistic nutrition approach, the results you experience can be profound in slimming yourself naturally.

You require learning just how to incorporate these 2 types of essential fats into your daily health lifestyle because there are a number of key essential fats that your body requires in balance and in proper ratios. I can provide you the knowledge of how to do this for your unique body constitution.

Be aware that everyone is unique so therefore you require learning how to structure your nutrition intake and how to input the proper fats and in the proper quantities for your unique body constitution. It is simply something you require to experience to see and feel the difference of when you have the proper holistic nutrition intake each day. You can visit my website to learn more about my services and my coaching programs that teach you how to structure your nutrition holistically and the proper use of essential fats. Go to www.MyBodyBrilliance.com

# Chapter 3

## Your Body Is A Sacred Temple

Your body is a Sacred Temple and is the most amazing creation in the entire Universe. If you only knew just how many biological processes your body is performing each second, you would marvel in awe each day. And, if you knew just how intelligent your body is and how it is able to manage and keep order of the billions of biological functions it requires to simply keep you alive.

Your body is by far the most amazing creation in the entire Universe. You will not find another creation in all of the Universe that is so complex and awesome as your body and how it is able to do all that it does each day. No computer could ever come close to doing what the body does. In fact, your body is processing more information in each second than thousands of advanced computers.

So, the holistic science of your body is that it requires basic foundational bio-nutrients each day as to be able to use as fuel to perform the many biological functions it does. When the body receives these vital life giving bio-nutrients, then it is able to function optimally. However, if you do not supply your body with these life giving bio-nutrients each day as is Divinely Intended to, then your body begins to function at reduced capacities and your ability to be healthy begins to be less. As such, the body begins to perform inefficiently and the homeostasis is off key.

When the body does not receive its foundational bio-nutrients on a consistent basis then you are setting yourself up for many health dis-functions due to your system not having the proper inputs to provide the necessary compounds to fuel your body. This is the case with many people in today's society. They are not inputting the proper nutrition on a consistent basis as to provide the body with its daily requirements. Thus, you get what you got with so many people being overweight and not healthy as they are not inputting viable holistic nutrition.

So, there are 2 main reasons why most people are not supplying their body with the proper inputs each day. One is that the food supply simply does not contain the hundreds of viable and life giving bio-nutrients that your body requires to function at peak capacity. What most people are unaware of is that a majority of the food supply is devoid of the hundreds of vital bio-nutrients that you require for optimal health. **This is due mainly because the modern agricultural practices have literally removed the healthy bio fauna in the form of living bacteria and fungi or what some call living probiotics.**

These little bacteria are the True Creators of the

hundreds of vital bio-nutrients that your body requires for optimum health. The modern agricultural practices are very unhealthy and have altered the soil ecology and as such you now have soils that are depleted and do not contain the living probiotics that are Divinely Designed to create the hundreds of life giving compounds for health and wellness for your body.

This is a BIG reason why so many people are not doing well these days. Most people are ingesting foods that are devoid of sound holistic nutrition. Your body can only go so long without its hundreds of life giving nutrient supply. The body eventually goes into survival mode and then begins to alter your hormone system. And by the way, hormones govern your metabolism which has the duty of converting food into usable foundational compounds that your body uses as fuel. When your body goes into survival mode it begins to lower your metabolic rate and essentially begins to burn calories slower. This is a natural survival mechanism of your body. It is designed to keep you alive.

**The issue with so many people today is that they are not supplying their body each day with the hundreds of vital bio-nutrients and the body has gone into survival mode.**

As such, their hormone system is off key and then alters the metabolism to burn calories slower as the body thinks it is not being fed. Simply know that just because you ingest a food, does not mean that it is going to nourish your system. In the case with modern produce, most of it is deficient in nutrition so even though you may ingest it, this does mean you are nourishing your body. In fact, the way most people go at nutrition, is that they are actually depleting their body by ingesting nutrient devoid foods.

It takes energy and enzymes and other bio-nutrients to break food into usable compounds by your cells. If the food you ingest does not have the hundreds of vital bio-nutrients then you are using up valuable energy, enzymes and other foundational reserve nutrients of your body for no purpose other than digesting the devoid compounds. So, you are actually depleting your system by consistently ingesting nutrient devoid food.

Many people think that ingesting organic produce is a better choice for receiving more nutrition. Well, actually, organic produce also does not contain the hundreds of vital bio-nutrients that you require to be healthy. Again, it is the modern agricultural practices that have altered the soil ecology and the probiotics.

So, organic produce usually is not going to be the solution as many people think. What requires to be corrected is the soil ecology and the natural vital probiotics. Get the probiotics back into the soil and now you can supply your body with its requirements. The only issue with this is that it costs quite a bit of money to get the probiotics at optimal levels.

So, as you can see this is quite an issue that requires to be addressed soon because your body can only go so long without receiving its hundreds of foundational nutrient supply. At some point the body begins to break down and you set yourself up for many health dis-functions.

What I am presenting is simple holistic science. This is something you can easily observe and validate. So now you have one of the main reasons as to why so many people are unhealthy and overweight. The food supply simply does not contain what is supposed to be there and as such the human body cannot function at peak levels. This is why it is essential for you to learn how to structure your nutrition holistically as to increase your vital nutrient intake.

Another main reason why so many people are unhealthy and overweight is that many foods available in grocery stores are processed and contain toxic ingredients in them. Even so called health foods that you can find at health food stores are not what is being claimed. You require being more discerning about what you believe as companies are putting flashy labels on their products claiming "healthy" yet if you learn the holistic science of what ingredients they are inputting into their foods then you will discover something that is not healthy.

You must be aware that processed foods are not ideal nutrition for the body. They are altered from their Divine state and as such they can no longer feed and nourish your body properly. Here is a simple formula so that you can comprehend the simple holistic science of health and your body.

**Your body is Divinely intended to be nourished via Mother Earth pure foods**.

Foods from nature in their natural state are the ideal form of nutrition for your body. It is this simple. You cannot outdo nature by creating processed food compounds and expect to be healthy.

Simply look at life and society and there have many people who are depleted and malnourished. It does not matter if you fill your belly. The main point is your body requires viable nutrition in the form of Mother Earth foods. This is simple holistic science. When you go to the gas station to fill up your gas tank, you get the right octane gas, correct? You wouldn't input a compound like kerosene or diesel in there would you? That would totally mess up your car.

Yet, this is what a majority of people are doing each day through the food choices they make. They do not comprehend that it is not as simple as ingesting any food compound to satisfy your hunger. You require nourishing your body with the vital hundreds of bio-nutrients that are essential for health and wellness.

A majority of the food supply is altered from its Divine state and cannot sustain life for long. **Just so you know is that most of the food supply is now either GMO**

**or hybridized forms of produce.** These altered forms of food cannot sustain human life for long. Your body simply cannot recognize the makeup due to the altering of the molecules of these food compounds. It is at the molecular level that your body breaks foods into and if you have a compound that is altered then your body will not recognize it as is Divinely intended to.

So, our society requires to wake up and learn the holistic science of health and then begin to restructure their nutrition intake as to supply the body with what is Divinely intended to feed and nourish it.

A byproduct of ingesting altered and processed foods is that it can cause the body to become toxic and depleted. For some it can actually cause weight gain as the body simply cannot process all of the toxic compounds from the foods they are ingesting. Your body requires many bio-nutrients to cleanse and detox your body of bio-wastes and other bio-toxins. If you are not supplying your body with its vital requirements then it simply cannot purge the toxic compounds out of your system. As such, you have accumulations of these bio-wastes and bio-toxins and then the body will store them in various place around the body. In fact, your body must now protect your system from these toxic compounds and thus it produces fat globules around them to neutralize them so they cannot cause any harm to your vital organs.

This is what is going on with many people in society. Their bodies are extremely toxic and depleted and the body has accumulated many bio-wastes and other toxins and now they are overweight because the body does not have the energy, enzymes and other detox compounds to keep the body clean and slim. Thus, you have an overweight society that is also depleted of energy as their system is not receiving the vital bio-nutrients that create energy and vitality.

Are you beginning to see the dilemma of the health of

society? It is not as simple as eating a little better and drinking more water. In fact, I will get into the water dilemma later. You must learn the holistic foundation that I am teaching, otherwise, you will be wasting time, money and energy. Most of the current health paradigms have no clue of these Truths I am presenting. They are teaching philosophies that are erroneous and in some cases counter health.

You must be careful as to what you believe especially with all of the health information out there. It is wild sea of information and most of it is not going to even come close to providing you the holistic foundation so you may be as healthy as possible.

As you can see by now there are a number of issues that require to be addressed otherwise more and more people will become overweight and unhealthy. The time has come for a Higher pathway for optimum health. This pathway is now here and I am presenting it in a manner that is simple and yet profound. The pathway I teach is based on holistic science and honors nature and your unique constitution of mind, body and spirit.

## Chapter 4

## The Truth About Sugar

Sugar is by far the unhealthiest compound for the human body. It does so many negative things to your body. If you truly knew just how unhealthy sugar is to your entire physiology, you would never touch the stuff ever again. Let me present some basic holistic science perspectives on sugar and why it is the unhealthiest compound for your health and your evolution.

You see, sugar is a processed compound. At the fundamental level sugar cane is taken from nature, stripped of its healthy components and then you are left with an altered compound that is toxic to your system and can do so many other negative things to affect your health. Sugar stimulates your nervous system and impacts your brain chemistry. It will actually make your brain become addicted to it and cause your brain to fire your neurons and neurotransmitters way too fast for health and wellness. Your neurotransmitters are there to relay information to many parts of the body for optimum functioning.

If you ingest sugar frequently, it will jack up your nervous system and then impact these transmitters to relay information too fast or imbalanced and thus you cannot have a calm physiology. Your brain body connection then gets thrown off and you have inefficient timing of information and relay of other vital communication between brain and body parts.

Ingesting sugar is also depleting to your system as it is not giving you energy as you think it may be. The energy you feel after ingesting sugar is your nervous system that has become stimulated and jacked up artificially. It is not pure energy and thus after some time, after the stimulation has worn off, your energy levels go way down. This is not healthy and is not the way nature intended for you and your health.

Sugar will also make your body acidic by lowering your body ph. If you comprehend anything about body ph, is that your body ph requires being within a specific range, otherwise, you set yourself up for many health disorders. Once your body ph has been lowered, there are now many factors that can cause you many health dis-functions.

Sugar also induces parasites and yeast in your body as many of these parasites thrive in an overly acidic internal body environment. You have many people nowadays who have yeast conditions and other parasitic causes and the link is usually sugar. As long as you are ingesting sugar in any of its processed forms, you set yourself up for parasites. As long as you have parasites in your system, you cannot be optimally healthy, not even close my friend.

Sugar is toxic to your system and can also put your body in survival mode. As such, your body will become toxic and thus it must protect your vital organ components. Thus, your body may actually produce fat globules around these toxins and now you set yourself up for weight gain. Sugar will also disrupt your liver function and metabolism because it will have a direct effect on your hormones.

Due to sugar being so toxic and stimulating to your system, it can cause your hormones to be thrown off key. Hormones govern your metabolism and thus you alter your metabolism by ingesting too much sugar or starchy food products.

Sweetened drinks are the worst compound to ingest as they profoundly alter your inner ph and physiology. This in turn can alter your hormones and eventually your metabolism. The drinks with corn syrup and other sweeteners in society that are so popular will cause you more weight gain and faster than anything else. My recommendation is stay away from all sweetened drinks, eve natural and organic juices and teas. These drinks are way too concentrated and can really mess up your hormones and physiology. It is not worth it.

Sodas are by far the worst sweetened drink as they have many negative factors as in they are loaded with sugar, they have phosphorous which is very acidic to your body and the carbonation is also a very acidic compound to your body. This makes this kind of drink a super unhealthy compound that has many negative implications to your health and well-being.

## Sugar Impacts Your Evolution Negatively

Ingesting sugar can also stifle your Higher Faculties of Intuition and other Spiritual Abilities. Its impact on the brain is very unhealthy and causes the brain chemistry to be thrown way off. As I explained, your brain is functioning at a multi-dimensional level and processing Higher Dimensional information along with governing your entire body physiology. Ingesting sugar essentially does not allow your brain to connect to your Higher Faculties which you require to evolve yourself.

To evolve you require to be tapped into your Higher Faculties of Intuition and other Higher Faculties. With sugar in your diet, you are doing a great disservice to your body and also to your evolution. Here is the main reason: **Your cells and DNA are supposed to be vibrating at faster than the speed of light.** Yes this is a fact! If you truly comprehend just how complex your body is and how many biological processes are occurring in each second then you will see that having your cells vibrating at the speed of light or lower is too slow for your body to function optimally.

You see, your cells require information in a steady

stream of pulsing energies or what some call Chi. In essence, your entire physiology is running via energy in the form of information coming from your brain as a direct link from Universal Consciousness or Source. The speed at which this happens is way beyond the speed of light, in fact probably a multiple thereof. It has to be at this super-fast speed in order for your entire body cellular system to receive all of the vast quantity of information coming in.

Here is a secret for you: When the cells and DNA of the body vibrate slower than the speed of light, this is when health disorders begin to set in. The relay of vital information your cells require to function optimally is simply too slow for your major systems to keep everything flowing as is Divinely intended.

Picture your wireless internet connection and when things are ideal you have super-fast loading and processing and everything is good. However, what happens if your internet connection begins to get bogged down and your computer starts to slow up and you cannot even load websites or check email. You have had this happen before and it makes your internet experience not fun.

Well, this is what happens when your body, cells and DNA are vibrating below the speed of light. Your cells simply cannot function as they are supposed to as the relay of vital energy and information that each cells requires is way too slow for optimum functioning. Do you see this? I pray you do because maybe, just maybe, you will begin to change your perspective on your health and your body?

**Ingesting sugar literally slows the vibration of your cells and DNA below the speed of light and thus sets you up for low level health.**

By the way, your DNA is so much more than some base nucleotides as modern science says. Your DNA is multi-dimensional and is also processing information from Source. There are components to DNA that cannot been seen by human eyes or microscopes, however, if you truly comprehend what DNA really is and what it really is doing you would marvel. Your DNA is actually like a multi-dimensional super computer and is constantly changing.

How does it change you may ask? It changes as you change. It changes with every thought you have, with every mood you have, it changes with what is going on in your environment as in the space you live and where you work. Do you comprehend what this means?

My friend, your DNA is constantly changing based on the frequencies and energies you are supplying it with via your thoughts, emotions, nutrition, your home environment, your work place, your friends, the music you listen to, the tv programs you watch, the clothes you wear and even the people you live with.

Maybe this is the motivation you require to do a

complete holistic lifestyle makeover? Until you understand life on this profound level as I am presenting to you then you will probably not make the changes in your life to experience shifts that will catapult your evolution.

This is why what I teach about holistic living is so profound, because it helps you to shift at the most profound levels and ensures you only input healthy frequencies and energies in, on and around your body as to help you to experience Higher levels of health and wellness. My friend, it is the only way for you to even begin to tap into your Higher Potentials.

**In essence, your body and your level of health is a direct link to your evolution as a human being and for being able to tap into your Higher Potentials.**

The healthier you are, the more you can tap into Higher Faculties and Higher Gifts and Talents as they will be able to come through since your cells and DNA are vibrating at faster than speed of light. Thus, Higher Dimensional information will be able to be processed by your brain and thus allow you to perform and do things that most people simply cannot do.

You will surprised to see just how much better you feel by simply removing all forms of processed sugar from your diet. In fact, within a few days you will feel a new sense of relief and calm and well-being.

There are many other food items that will have similar physiological effects on your body as sugar does. Most people are simply unaware that everything you ingest breaks down into smaller components. Many food items that people ingest actually will break down into sugar-like compounds.

Food items such as white flour products, white rice, cereal, potato chips, pretzels, corn chips, crackers and other dry brittle food items will get converted into sugar once in your body. As such, the physiological effect is that these food items can actually cause you to gain weight due to the effect on your metabolism and inefficient functioning of your entire biological system. These processed food items are not nutrition for your body and will only serve to lower your level of health. My recommendation is to stay away from these food items as there are far healthier alternatives.

I have written a recipe called **Fun Food Fantastic** that has some of the most knock your socks off meal creations. I have in the recipe book super delicious and healthy recipes that will satisfy your taste buds and be healthy for your body. You can go to Amazon.com or my website www.MyBodyBrilliance.com to download it.

# Chapter 5

## Holistic Nutrition Is Designed For Your Body

Holistic nutrition is what is supposed to go in your body. It is this simple. Put into your body what is supposed to go in there and now you can create optimum health. The issue of today and modern living is that convenience has taken priority over sound nutrition and as such you have many health issues. If you truly desire to be healthy and slim then you must learn this holistic nutrition pathway as it will be a much more efficient and healthier approach to living a healthy and happy life.

If you are healthy then it translates you into being happier which then affects other areas of your life. It is all connected my friend.

**Your health is your foundation for your life. With optimum health, you can go out into the world and do amazing things. You can inspire people by simply being slim, healthy and radiant. It is a choice only you can make.**

How much longer do you want to continue to be unhealthy, overweight or out of shape? It is not fun, is it? Just imagine how great you will feel by being slim and healthy. Imagine all of the activities that you can do and imagine when you go shopping for clothes how much of a happier process that will be by being able to purchase clothing that is in reduced sizes and fit you nicely. You can be slim and healthy my friend. The question is…**Are You Ready To Walk The Holistic Pathway That Will Get You There?**

# Chapter 6

## Your Multi-Dimensional Self

You see, you are comprised of a multi-dimensional complex that makes up your individual expression of who you are. You are a physical, mental, emotional and spiritual being in one. As such, you require comprehending that your health is a combination of the balance in these levels of your being. All of these are connected and it is like a pond where if you throw a rock into the pond, there is a ripple that emanates out to affect the entire pond.

Well, your physical, mental, emotional and spiritual constitution functions in the similar manner. If something affects you on one level it automatically ripples and affects the others.

Many people have mental, emotional and spiritual issues and thus this will eventually affect you physically. What has been discovered by numerous professional fields is that your mental, emotional and spiritual well-being have more of a pull on your health than do physical factors.

In fact, I feel that your level of health is about 3/4 attributed to your mental, emotional and spiritual balance and only about 1/4 due to physical factors. Many people could easily become healthier if they would begin to resolve these mental, emotional and spiritual imbalances.

Picture your car with 4 wheels. Now, in order for you to drive straight and smoothly, you require all four tires inflated to proper measures and also balanced. What would happen if one or more of your car tires was inflated improperly? Or, what do you think would happen if you had one or more flat tires on your car? You would not be able to drive straight let alone go anywhere if you have one or more flat tires.

Most of society is attempting to go at health with literally one wheel on their car of life. Most people do not know how to care for their mental, emotional or spiritual components to their being. As such, you have many people living imbalanced lives and have many health issues.

It has been shown that many people who are overweight have subconscious factors that are actually the root cause for a person's body storing fat and make them overweight. In fact, mind science research clearly validates that subconscious beliefs and disharmonies can cause a person to have unconscious motives to be large and overweight as to protect them from getting hurt.

Being overweight or fat is a buffer if you will as to keep people away as to not allow them to get too close. Your subconscious mind can do all sorts of things based on the beliefs you carry and the perspective you have about certain aspects of your life. Usually, very overweight people have inner subconscious disharmonies that are the True contributing factor to their condition.

So, if you truly desire to be healthy and slim, then you require learning how to nourish your multi-dimensional self. All aspects of your being comprise your health so don't you think it is about time you learn how to do this for yourself as to create a holistic foundation that gets you results? By beginning to balance and heal your mental, emotional and spiritual complex, you make it much easier for you to be physically healthy and slim. The results speak for themselves.

# Chapter 7

## Evolution Is The Only Goal of Life

So, if you look at the issues I presented earlier which are mainly physical then there is a byproduct of those effects. In this case, because your body is not receiving its requirements each day then this will eventually affect you mentally and emotionally and then spiritually.

What I am about to present is only known by a few people on the planet. Please listen carefully as this is a profound revelation and it has monumental proportions. If you do not supply the body with its daily requirements there are now implications that impact your evolution as a spiritual being. You see, your brain and mind are linked at the fundamental level.

Your brain is the super computer of your entire physiology and is the master control system for telling everything in your body to do what it does. In order for it to do this, it must have energy in the form of vital bio-nutrients that contain viable life force energy. Without these vital bio-nutrients and the life force energy that surrounds those nutrients, your brain simply cannot function as it is Divinely supposed to.

In essence, your entire biological physiology will become imbalanced. Your Higher Faculties will also not be able to come through which is your link to Universal Intelligence or what some call intuition or your connection to Source.

There are specific bio-nutrients that your brain requires to be able to process Higher Dimensional information. Do you comprehend how important this is? Essentially, you can increase your connection to Source by ingesting holistic nutrition and being as healthy as possible. This is about your evolution as a human being and is the most important aspect to your life. You are here to evolve your being my friend. You can only do that if you are as healthy as possible. You can only do that if you are supplying your body with what it requires to plug you into Source and your Higher Faculties.

Essentially, you can easily expand your consciousness by being healthy and ingesting Divine nutrition from Mother Earth and drinking structured water as nature intended. It is the way it has been designed my friend. Do you see the Sacred Truth of what I am presenting? This is simple holistic science and a majority of humanity simply does not know this Truth.

**A healthy society is conducive to evolution and a harmonic living environment.**

What you see in society today is largely in part due to the inappropriate structuring of viable nutrition for human health. Healthy people are much nicer and calmer and more balanced than people who ingest toxic and unhealthy nutrition. Healthy people have more creative ideas and do amazing things in life. They are much happier and usually have a passion for helping people.

Healthy people are supplying their body with the vital life force energy in the form of Mother Earth foods as to create a stronger connection to Source and their Intuition and Higher Faculties. Viable nutrition has the direct capacity to impact your moods as well, as your brain can then create the necessary electrical synapse functions as to produce the life enhancing hormones and neuro-transmitters.

**Yes, my friend, sound holistic nutrition can bliss you out if you know how to structure your daily nutrition in a balanced form.**

As you can see, your nutrition intake can significantly impact your moods and your mental and emotional well-being. And in turn, this will eventually affect you spiritually as in your Higher Faculties for your evolution.

So, this is why I teach what I teach. I want you to know that your health is your foundation to life. It is your link to your evolution. I am here to provide you a fresh holistic pathway that can impact you on many levels of your being as to help you evolve your being while you are on this planet.

## Chapter 8

## Sacred Water & Its Link To Your Health and Evolution

I think you know just how important water is to your health. However, what you probably do not know is that your body requires a specific type of water for optimum health. You see, simply drinking water is not necessarily going to benefit your health and well-being. There are a number of reasons as to why there is an issue with most of the water supply on planet earth.

First, is that as a human being, you are meant to be drinking water from nature as in running streams and rivers. This is how is how it was Divinely intended to be from the beginning of time and as long as humans have been around. Water from nature is in a perfect Sacred state that impacts your health in profound ways. You see, water is meant to serve 3 functions. One, water's main function is to transport viable bio-nutrients to the cell membrane where receptor sites for each nutrient are.

The second function for water is to enter the cell and cleanse any bio-wastes that may be there. And third, the gases of water have some biological function in the cell as to provide energy when the oxygen and hydrogen molecules are split apart. In totality, water is a main provider of energy for your body. It is meant to keep you healthy and young and radiant.

However, the water supply of today simply does not have these Divine qualities any longer. Water has become altered from its Divine state and thus can no longer provide you the life giving qualities that it is Divinely intended to. You may think that bottled water or filtered water is good for your health? Well, let me clarify some basic holistic science on water that has many implications for your health and well-being.

The molecular structure to Sacred water or water from nature as in rivers and streams is unique and properly structured to be absorbed by your cells. The size of the molecules is also unique in natural Sacred water as to be able to enter through the cell aquaporin. Sacred water is also charged with life force energy from Mother Earth.

When you drink properly structured water, it instantly energizes your body and brings viable nutrients to your cells. Thus, water is the greatest nutrient and the quickest way to input energy into your body.

The issue with the current water supply is that it no

longer contains life force energy and the molecular size is too BIG to enter the aquaporin of the cell as processing water literally alters the Divine state. Bottled water is processed and is also acidic due to being in plastic. These both contribute to altering the waters' molecules and removing the life force energy. This kind of water is actually depleting to your system as it really cannot get into the aquaporin but also the acidity lowers your body ph which impacts your health in many negative ways.

So, the common filtering processes as in reverse osmosis, distillation and deionization and such actually make water unhealthy to drink long term as they make the water acidic and do not have the Sacred Molecular Structure that your body requires to be fully hydrated. These types of processed waters will deplete your system of viable nutrients and can cause issues with certain organs.

So now you have another issue with nourishing the body properly. As I spoke about earlier, the food supply is devoid of viable nutrition. Now throw on top of that water that cannot enter into the aquaporin of your cells due to the molecular size. This sets you up for major health disorders and malnourishment. Do you see this?

If you truly want to be healthy then you must start with your water supply. Water makes everything you do for health function at optimal levels. Water is also your link to your evolution. Your brain actually uses the most hydration of any organ or part of the body. When your brain does not receive adequate hydration each day, it simply cannot function at peak capacity and thus your link to Higher Faculties is lessened.

Think of your brain just like your car battery. In your car battery, there is water as to provide the proper electrical balance and induction to supply power. Without the proper amount of water in your car battery, you simply will not have juice or viable power to fuel your car. Well, your brain functions in the similar manner. It must have consistent supply of hydration as to provide the proper electrical balance to function multi-dimensionally. Yes, your brain is a multi-dimensional power house and it has so many functions.

Like I said, you would marvel if you truly knew just how amazing your body is and what is going on in each second. Your brain is performing billions of processes in a second and also processing Higher Dimensional frequencies and information as to help you be healthy and for your evolution. Do you see how profound this is?

**The fact is...most people are super dehydrated due to drinking non structured water and not supplying the body and brain with its requirements.**

The other important point is that you must have properly structured water each day as to purge the body of bio-wastes and other bio-toxins. If you do not, your body then begins to store these in various parts of the body and thus you set yourself up for weight gain and low level health. As I said earlier, your body will produce fat globules around toxins as to protect your organ systems.

Thus, many people are very toxic and carrying many pounds worth of accumulated bio-wastes and fat that surrounds those wastes. Look at society and there you have many people who have toxic systems. **Working out and doing cardio and limiting fat and calories is not a solution to this major health dis-function.** This is why the many diet programs and other so called weight reduction solutions have not worked universally to help people to get the excess weight off and keep it off.

**The solution lies in learning the holistic science of human health. This is the only way to structure your lifestyle and your nutrition as to provide you the foundation that is required for you to be healthy, slim and radiant.**

So, you can see by now that the current health issues in society are not some mystery. Society thinks it is, however, when you go to the core essence of life, there you have the Truth sitting there in front you. How many millions of people have missed what I am presenting I do not know. However, the time is at hand and there must be a profound shift in humanity's consciousness if we are going anywhere and do anything productive as a whole. The health of most humans requires being addressed and corrected.

**As a species we can only evolve when a majority of humans are healthy and happy.** It is this simple. So, if you want to create a harmonic planet, restore the nutrition and water supply and watch what happens and how quickly.

It is quite interesting that the 2 main vehicles for nourishing your body are not even close to being healthy or proper for your health. The mystery is over my friend. You now have in your consciousness the Truth of life's health issues. The solutions are quite simple if you are willing to walk the holistic path to health and wellness. Yes, it is going to require some effort and restructuring of your lifestyle and your consciousness, however, the benefits will be profound.

# Chapter 9

## The 5 Holistic Keys For Being Healthy & Slim

There are 5 main holistic keys that will ensure you stay healthy, slim and radiant throughout your life. These are foundational requirements and provide a sound structure as to live from. These keys are simple, yet profound and must be practiced consistently.

**# 1 - Stop Inputting The Grunge Foods Into Your Body Temple** – the first thing you can do to begin your path to a healthier and slimmer you is to stop inputting foods and compounds that are not meant to go in the human body. There are many and so you must learn what foods are healthy and which are not.

About 3/4 of the foods on grocery store shelves are not healthy or food for your body. A clue is anything that is in a box, a can or any package has been processed and is altered from its Divine state. Thus, it may not be a healthy choice for nutrition.

Just as when you gas up your car, you input the proper octane gas in there. Your body is probably billions of times more important than your car so just raise your consciousness and begin to treat your body as a Sacred Temple...because it is!!!

You can go to my website to download my Holistic Food Guide and Holistic Grocery List Guide as to help you with making healthier grocery choices. Go To www.MyBodyBrilliance.com

**#2 - Input Holistic Nutrition Into Your Body Temple** – put what is supposed to go into your body there. This means simple Mother Earth foods that are Divinely intended to nourish your body. This may sound simple and it is yet most people are simply not doing it on a daily basis. So, begin ingesting clean produce and ensure you eat 3 balanced and holistic meals per day. In my new book called

*Sensational Slimming Secrets: A Revolutionary Pathway To A Healthier & Slimmer You* I reveal the Holistic Formula that is universally effective for helping most people to slim themselves easily and naturally. This will be the greatest investment in your health and will supply you the holistic foundation as to help you to be slim and healthy for life. You can go to Amazon.com to purchase it or simply go to my website at RinoSoriano.com

**#3 - Cleanse Your Body Temple** – if you truly desire to be slim and healthy then you are going to require learning how to cleanse your body of all the accumulated bio-wastes, heavy metals, parasites and toxins from your entire system. This is the greatest process you can do for your health and well-being.

You have to comprehend that if you are toxic and have many years' worth of accumulated bio-wastes in your body, you cannot slim yourself. Your body simply will not let go of the fat since it is actually protecting your organs and other vital body components.

It is pointless to do fitness activities and diets as these are not the solution. Millions of people have attempted the common philosophies for weight reduction and you now actually have more people who are overweight. Not the path to take my friend. That is the hamster wheel approach and has proven to be super ineffective to helping people to reduce their weight. These paradigms are unnatural to human physiology and can actually deplete you of sound nutrition.

The LIMIT YOUR FAT & CALORIES paradigms are unhealthy, unwise and VERY INEFFECTIVE at reducing your weight. They actually cause you to alter your basal metabolic rate to burn calories slower as the body will go into survival mode since you are reducing too many healthy fats and calories your body requires for energy. This is counter-productive and the proof is simply look at society and see what these paradigms have gotten people. This approach makes people more overweight because it alters the metabolism in an unhealthy manner.

Cleansing your body in a holistic manner will begin to expel the bio-wastes and other toxins and will help with raising the energy levels of your system. As you continue to do this, now your body will begin to shed weight easily without reducing calories and pointless cardio activities.

There is a holistic process to go about this and I provide a holistic pathway that you simply follow. This is the greatest thing you can learn on your path to a healthier and slimmer you. You will be amazed at how easy slimming becomes when you learn this holistic cleansing and holistic nutrition structuring. You can visit my website to learn more about my cleaning programs at RinoSoriano.com

**#4 - Holistic Fitness: The Secret Holistic Process For Being Fit & Slim** – the fitness activities that most people are performing are not healthy as claimed. In fact, the common fitness activities can actually be counter-health. Once again, if you learn the holistic science of your body then you will come to discover that performing high intensity and long duration cardiovascular activities as commonly taught out there are unhealthy and not required to be fit and slim.

Your heart does not require the stimulation that cardiovascular activities supply. The last thing you want to do for your health is to stimulate your heart levels to high intensity like is being taught in society. This places unneeded strain on your heart and does not make you fit like you may think. **You do not get fit by doing any cardiovascular activities. This is a myth!**

Being fit is a direct reflection of how well your physiology and metabolism is functioning. It has nothing to do with how much cardiovascular training you do. That is a myth and is actually unhealthy for human health. Once again, if you simply look at holistic science then you will discover that doing any high intensity activity for long duration will cause your body to think it is in retreat mode and running from something.

This is a Divine natural mechanism as to protect you in case you require fleeing from something that is coming after you. Being that we no longer live in the wild, this mechanism usually is not functioning. However, by performing high intensity cardio activities you are placing your body in this mode without even knowing it.

Many people each day are wasting their energy by doing such activities as cardio machines, aerobics, tread mill, and running which is the most unhealthy activity as it is hard on the physical joints, tendons, ligaments and your entire physiology. Running degenerates the body and breaks muscle tissue down. It is counter health regardless of the claims in favor for it. All of these cardio activities are unneeded and unhealthy.

To get fit you must learn the holistic process for doing

so. I teach what is called holistic fitness and the results speak for themselves. **With holistic fitness, you actually save energy and only do activities that build muscle.** You do activities that do not stimulate your heart unnaturally.

**Holistic fitness is very efficient and results come very quickly**. Once you learn this holistic process for being fit, you will see how profound the benefits you receive. This is one of the greatest practices you can learn on your journey to a healthier and slimmer you. You can learn more about my holistic fitness programs on my website at RinoSoriano.com

**#5 - Balancing Your Mental, Emotional and Spiritual Constitution** - balancing and healing your mental, emotional and spiritual complex is probably the most important component to your health. These aspects to your being have a BIG pull on your physical health so it will be wise for you to begin to nurture and nourish these aspects to yourself. As you do, you may experience many shifts in your health and well-being and your desire for grunge foods may even subside. Many people resort to ingesting comfort foods when they experience rough times in their life. Most of the time these comfort foods are sugary and salty and processed as they appeal to the taste buds but not your body.

You can begin to heal and balance these aspects to your being by sitting with yourself each day and simply chill, relax, meditate and say affirmations out loud that are High Frequency. You do not always have to be doing something or talking.

In fact, you waste a lot of energy each day by talking too much and doing things just to be busy. You must chill and connect with these unseen parts to you, otherwise, you cannot be balanced and have harmony among your total wholeness.

It may be a good idea to hire a spiritual coach or mentor to help you with learning how to heal and calm your mental, emotional and spiritual complex. I do Consciousness Coaching and it is quite powerful as it goes to the core aspect of your life issue. It will be wise for you to begin to learn how to elevate your consciousness to resolve your life issues for yourself.

You will see and feel shifts in your being the more you make it a daily habit and practice of going within and giving yourself some love and nurturing. You can begin by treating yourself with love and honor and just appreciate who you are.

You can take some time each day to simply go into nature somewhere and simply sit and connect with Mother Earth and ground yourself. Mother Earth is very healing and by connecting to her you can help to heal your inner being.

Everyone requires inner balancing and inner nurturing of some kind so please begin to simply go out in nature and just connect. Sit on the grass, sit on the beach, go climb a tree, anything to connect you with nature. You will be surprised at the results of doing this simple and free practice consistently.

You can also write down any feelings you are having about any area of life and simply write down anything that comes up. Just get it out on paper and then burn it. Keep writing and let whatever come flow and then learn to say I Forgive You to whomever or whatever is bothering you. Use the following mantra to help you with creating more harmony in your life:

**I Love My Self and I Easily Forgive Everyone, Especially** _____ (fill in whomever is bothering you here or it can also be a specific situation, say it out loud and as many times as possible throughout the day)

What I have learned is having any anger, rage or resentment at anyone will set you up for many life challenges. The Universe will continue to send you challenging life situations until you surrender your anger, rage or resentment. Having any one of these toxic emotions literally affects your health and well-being and also other areas of your life as in relationships and even finances. You will be surprised to discover how when you can truly forgive someone how your life begins to improve and your health is better.

My friend, forgiveness is the Universal Elixir of life and at this time on this planet everyone could sure use a dose of this profound nectar of life. Forgiveness will literally set you free. If you have any negative feelings toward anyone it is best to begin doing forgiveness practices as to help you elevate your life. This can really elevate your health and wellness.

**Forgiveness Practice:**

Sit in a quiet place on a chair or even in nature in the grass, beach, or mountain. Close your eyes and call in the Creator, Your Spirit, Mother Earth and any other holy being that you feel connected to. Say: Dear Source, I am so sorry for anyone I have ever hurt at any time. Please forgive me for having done anything to anyone that caused them to feel hurt or harmed. I also ask that I be able to forgive anyone that has ever hurt me or caused me harm. I wish to forgive them unconditionally. Thank You!

This life can be challenging and sometimes you may feel overwhelmed, however, just know that everything will be ok. You must learn to forgive everyone in your life as they are only doing and being who they are. Yes, some people will simply treat you in a funny way or not honor you, however, the best motto is not to expect anything from anyone because they could never meet the expectations of your ego anyway. So, learn to let things go and just create a harmonic space for yourself in your home where it is to be your Sacred Sanctuary where nothing can bother you.

You may feel profound shifts in your health and other areas of your life as you begin to nurture your full being. So, give it a go and be sure to reach out for help if you require. Everyone can benefit from a coach to help make things more efficient and be there to support you. You can contact me for coaching or I can refer you to someone in my network that specializes with these topics.

## Chapter 10

### Your Mission As A Healthy Being

Ok, so I have given you more than enough to contemplate for now. The time has come for you to learn how to live a holistic lifestyle and how to structure your nutrition for optimum health. There is no one way to health as many people believe. There is no one magic diet or supplemental program that suits everyone. You require learning about your full constitution and then you begin to explore and structure your nutrition based on a holistic foundation with some feedback from your Intuition and Body Wisdom.

In essence, your health is individual unto you so it is best for you to discover the process for optimum health and being slim. This is the greatest investment for your entire life. Being healthy is a lifestyle and a decision you make from your heart. You cannot supplement your way to health as many people believe. Once again...Where is The Proof?

You can only get to optimum health and a slim you by embodying a holistic lifestyle foundation that serves you and your life and your unique mind, body, spirit complex. This is a process and only you can do it. What I have done is created a holistic pathway that anyone can follow and get results that last. It is like a roadmap that guides you to your desired destination. You require this holistic health roadmap if you truly desire to be healthy and slim for life.

So, the roadmap is here, now you simply just make a choice that you are going to walk this path to your desired destination. I will love to teach you and walk you down this holistic path if you are ready to step up to the plate and elevate your life and your health and slim your body.

Look, by you becoming slimmer and healthier you will open up a new world and a new life for yourself. You will be able to live life on a much Higher level and have excess energy. You will also feel more confident in yourself as looking healthy and slim automatically elevates your confidence. True confidence is a quality that can expand your life in quantum leaps. Confidence from within is how you can experience your full potential as a human being. Being healthy and slim is the confidence foundation that you require to go out in life and rock.

So, you now have a choice to make...you can continue to follow the many hamster wheel approaches to health and weight reduction or you can learn a holistic pathway that actually validates itself with results that you experience on the totality of your being. What are you going to choose my friend???

Here is what I believe. I feel that you owe it to yourself and the planet to be as healthy, fit and radiant as possible. **By being in this optimum state, you can then go out and do amazing things with your life because you will have the energy to do so and you will also have the creativity and motivation.** Also, by being healthy and radiant and slim, this is a pathway to your evolution as a human being. After all, this is the main goal of you being on this planet.

Do you really think you can evolve at full potential by being overweight and not feeling well? My friend, it is a dishonor to yourself and the planet by playing life small and being unhealthy and out of shape. Why would you even consider living life at this level? Please step up to the plate and begin your journey to a healthier and slimmer you. If you truly want to help this Sacred Planet evolve and be more harmonic then you have a huge impact on that.

You can help thousands of people simply by being healthy, slim and radiant by being an example of what is possible for a human. You will also inspire others to want to be healthy and slim like you. You can serve as the catalyst for many people waking up and living a holistic lifestyle that benefits everyone. Everything is going there anyway, so simply do it for the entire planet. You must make this about the entire planet because if you make this just about yourself, you will not have enough motivation to be 100% in.

Think of it as a mission of monumental proportions that has profound implications as to help this planet to heal and create harmony and peace for all. What if the fate of humanity and the planet rested on your shoulders? What if how healthy you are and what lifestyle you live impacts many thousands of people? What if by being healthy and slim you actually help save this planet and the future of humans? **Well, I must inform you then that the fate of humanity does rest on your shoulders!!!**

Your health and your evolution are a direct way you can help this planet to heal. By making the decision right now to begin your holistic lifestyle makeover, you set a ripple in play that can go out and affect many people on the planet. And then they can set another ripple that affects many others as well. Do you see the profundity of this? Do you comprehend how important it is for you to be healthy and slim?

**A healthy and radiant and happy society creates harmony and peace and well-being.** These are natural byproducts of healthy people.

So, please make the decision today to step up to the plate and do your part to help yourself be healthier and slimmer and set the ripple that can impact many, many people. I think everyone on this planet owes it to Mother Earth and humanity to be as healthy and radiant as possible as this translates into many beautiful experiences.

I wish you many blessings on your holistic lifestyle makeover.

To Your Health,

Rino Soriano

**Revolutionary Entrepreneur**
**Empath Alignment Mentor**
**Life Force Catalyst**
**Holistic Nutrition Consultant**
**Holistic Fitness Coach**
**Holistic Chef**

**Here are Rino's other life transforming books:**

**Body Brilliance,** The 8 Royal Diamonds For A Healthier and More Radiant You

**Fun Food Fantastic,** Knock Your Socks Off Meal Creations

**Mystic Smoothies,** The 33 Most Delicious and Nutritious Smoothies To Rock The Planet

**Youngevity Revolution,** The 12 Secret Spirals To Enduring Youth and Longevity

**Sensational Slimming Secrets,** A Revolutionary Pathway To A Healthier & Slimmer You

**Acne Busters,** How To Vaporize Acne in 3 Weeks or Less

**Wart Busters,** How To Vaporize Warts in 3 Weeks

**Bodybuilding Brilliance**, Massive Muscle Makeover

**Sports Brilliance,** A Revolutionary Pathway To Your Higher Sports Performance

You may visit Rino's website to learn more about his coaching programs, holistic recipes, videos and for upcoming live transformational events. You can visit at RinoSoriano.com

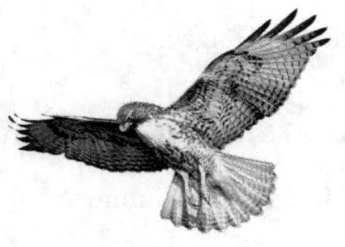

www.ingramcontent.com/pod-product-compliance
Lightning Source LLC
Chambersburg PA
CBHW060202290526
45789CB00003B/1131

*  9 7 8 1 5 0 1 0 6 8 7 3 7  *